Contents

Acknowledgments *iv*

The Case for Carbohydrate Counting *1*

Carbohydrate Counting Defined *2*

Who Should Learn Carbohydrate Counting? *2*

Educator Skills and Time *4*

Helpful Carbohydrate Counting Teaching Tools *5*

Basic Carbohydrate Counting *6*

The Nuts and Bolts *6*

Case Studies *15*

Advanced Carbohydrate Counting *21*

The Nuts and Bolts *21*

Case Studies *32*

Advanced Carbohydrate Counting Using an Insulin Pump *37*

The Nuts and Bolts *37*

Case Study *38*

Special Considerations and Situations *42*

Access to Diabetes Educators/Registered Dietitians *48*

References *49*

Appendices *51*

1. Glycemic Control for People with Diabetes *51*

2. How Much Carbohydrate to Eat and When? *52*

3. Carbohydrate Counting Resources *53*

4. Record Keeping Form *55*

5. Carbohydrate Counting Teaching Checklist *56*

6. How Much Carbohydrate Is Needed? *57*

Index *58*

Acknowledgments

We are pleased to provide this much-needed practical guide on teaching carbohydrate counting. We hope it will be a valuable resource for health care professionals teaching carbohydrate counting and that, ultimately, it will help people with diabetes achieve their desired level of glycemic control. The content presented in this guide has evolved over the years with the input and expertise of many of our colleagues, including: Betty Brackenridge, MS, RD, CDE; Anne Daly, MS, RD, CDE; Paul Davidson, MD; James A. Dicke, MD; Sandy Gillespie, RD, CDE; Karmeen Kulkarni, MS, RD, CDE; James H. Mersey, MD, FACP, FACE; and Thomas J. Sporney, RPh. Countless other colleagues and people with diabetes have contributed to the state of the art of carbohydrate counting, and we are indebted to them as well.

We also thank our colleagues who graciously provided their expertise and time by reviewing this practical guide: Dianne Davis, RD, LDN, CDE; Sandy Gillespie, RD, CDE; Janie Lipps, MSN, RN-C, CDE; Pat Richardson, RN, MN, NP; and John Walsh, PA, CDE.

Last, we are indebted to Christine Welch, Associate Director, Professional Books, American Diabetes Association, for her vision in recognizing the need for this practical guide and for her editorial expertise from beginning to end.

PRACTICAL
Carbohydrate
Counting

A How-to-Teach Guide for Health Professionals

Hope S. Warshaw, MMSc, RD, CDE
Karen M. Bolderman, RD, LD, CDE

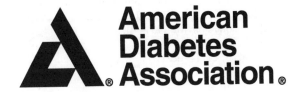

American Diabetes Association®

Director, Book Publishing, John Fedor; *Associate Director, Professional Books,* Christine B. Welch; *Production Manager,* Peggy M. Rote; *Composition and Text Design,* Circle Graphics, Inc.; *Cover Design,* Bremmer & Goris Communications; *Printer,* Transcontinental Printing, Inc.

Printed in Canada
1 3 5 7 9 10 8 6 4 2

The suggestions and information contained in this publication are generally consistent with the *Clinical Practice Recommendations* and other policies of the American Diabetes Association, but they do not represent the policy or position of the Association or any of its boards or committees. Reasonable steps have been taken to ensure the accuracy of the information presented. However, the American Diabetes Association cannot ensure the safety or efficacy of any product or service described in this publication. Individuals are advised to consult a physician or other appropriate health care professional before undertaking any diet or exercise program or taking any medication referred to in this publication. Professionals must use and apply their own professional judgment, experience, and training and should not rely solely on the information contained in this publication before prescribing any diet, exercise, or medication. The American Diabetes Association—its officers, directors, employees, volunteers, and members—assumes no responsibility or liability for personal or other injury, loss, or damage that may result from the suggestions or information in this publication.

⊗ The paper in this publication meets the requirements of the ANSI Standard Z39.48-1992 (permanence of paper).

ADA titles may be purchased for business or promotional use or for special sales. For information, please write to Lee Romano Sequeira, Special Sales & Promotions, at the address below.

American Diabetes Association
1701 North Beauregard Street
Alexandria, Virginia 22311

Library of Congress Cataloging-in-Publication Data

Warshaw, Hope S., 1954–
    Practical carbohydrate counting : a how-to-teach guide for health professionals / Hope S. Warshaw, Karen M. Bolderman.
      p. cm.
    Includes index.
    ISBN 1-58040-123-6 (pbk. : alk. paper)
    1. Diabetics—Nutrition—Study and teaching. 2. Diabetes—Diet therapy—Study and teaching. 3. Food—Carbohydrate content—Study and teaching. 4. Patient education. I. Bolderman, Karen M., 1954– II. Title.
    RC662 .W3153 2001
    616.4'620654'071—dc21

                                           2001040047

The Case for Carbohydrate Counting

Carbohydrate counting is a popular meal planning approach for several reasons. First, excellent blood glucose goals can be achieved with carbohydrate counting. Large-scale clinical trials, specifically the Diabetes Control and Complications Trial (DCCT)(1) and United Kingdom Prospective Diabetes Study (2), have provided unequivocal evidence for the important of glycemic control in preventing and delaying diabetes complications. In the DCCT, carbohydrate counting was used as one of four meal planning approaches and found to be effective in helping people achieve glycemic control while allowing flexibility in their food choices (3). In support of the imperative of glycemic control, the American Diabetes Association (ADA) position statement "Nutrition Recommendations and Principles for People with Diabetes Mellitus" cites maintenance of near-normal blood glucose levels as the number one priority (4). See ADA's goals for glycemic control for people with diabetes in Appendix 1. In addition, monitoring postprandial blood glucose levels (PPG), defined as two hours after the start of a meal (5), provides valuable information with which to teach and fine-tune the skills of carbohydrate counting.

Second, as we have learned more about the impact of carbohydrate on blood glucose levels, we better understand how to intervene. Carbohydrate is the primary nutrient that raises PPG. Carbohydrate begins to raise blood glucose within 15 minutes after initiation of food intake and is converted to nearly 100% glucose within about two hours. This is not true for the other three calorie-containing nutrients, protein, fat, and alcohol. The ADA nutrition recommendations encourage a focus on total carbohydrate intake rather than differentiating between types of carbohydrates. "Although various starches do have different glycemic responses, from a clinical perspective, first priority should be given to the total amount of carbohydrate consumed rather than the source of the carbohydrate."(4)

Third, carbohydrate counting is an easy meal planning approach for health care professionals to teach and for people to learn. The focus of carbohydrate counting is on the one nutrient that most impacts blood glucose. People can learn to relate their carbohydrate intake with their blood glucose results. People are encouraged by the flexibility and practical nature of carbohydrate counting and enjoy including foods they regularly consume, such as convenience and restaurant foods. Carbohydrate counting is the meal planning approach that most closely aligns with both today's diabetes management goals and the lifestyle and food habits of many people.

Although carbohydrate counting is a relatively easy meal planning approach for health professionals to teach and for people to learn, the reality is that the implementation and effective use of any type of diabetes meal planning requires time and energy from the person with diabetes as well as the health professionals involved with their care.

CARBOHYDRATE COUNTING DEFINED

Carbohydrate counting is really two meal-planning approaches of differing complexity. In basic carbohydrate counting, goals are to draw attention to the foods that contain carbohydrate, and to encourage people to eat consistent amounts of carbohydrate at meals and snacks (if necessary or desired) at similar times each day. Advanced carbohydrate counting is appropriate for people who use multiple daily injections (MDI) of insulin or continuous subcutaneous insulin infusion (CSII) via an insulin pump. Their goal is to learn to match the amount of rapid- (lispro or aspart) or short-acting (regular) insulin they take with or before eating to the amount of carbohydrate they choose to eat. They use an insulin:carbohydrate ratio, which is calculated based on individual insulin needs and metabolic responses to carbohydrate. It is essential to master basic carbohydrate counting to become proficient at advanced carbohydrate counting.

WHO SHOULD LEARN CARBOHYDRATE COUNTING?

Carbohydrate counting is appropriate for people of all ages and all types of diabetes—type 1, type 2, or gestational diabetes. Carbohydrate counting can be individualized to fit any stage of life (6–11).

- Consider the young child with type 1 diabetes whose appetite is unpredictable. The parents might find it helpful to use an individualized insulin:carbohydrate ratio to provide the appropriate amount of rapid-acting insulin when the meal is complete and the amount of carbohydrate consumed is known.
- Consider the older person with type 2 on one oral diabetes medication who wants an easy-to-follow structured plan. This person can be taught to eat a certain amount of carbohydrate at meals and be provided with a few sample meals to meet the recommended amount of carbohydrate.

Generally, basic carbohydrate counting is most appropriate for people with type 2 diabetes who control their diabetes with a healthy eating plan and physical activity with or without the addition of oral diabetes agents. It is also a good starting point for people with type 2 on insulin or a combination of insulin and oral diabetes medications as well as people with type 1 diabetes who use a conventional insulin regimen (2–3 injections per day), MDI, or a pump. People who use MDI or a pump will likely want to progress to advanced carbohydrate counting to help them achieve greater glycemic control and take advantage of the flexibility their insulin regimen is designed to provide.

Beyond considerations of the type of diabetes and management regimen the person follows, as with any meal planning approach, success will be based on the person's individual ability and willingness to follow guidelines and level of motivation to achieve glycemic control. For basic carbohydrate counting, a person must have the ability to

- perform simple addition and subtraction
- read and use the Nutrition Facts found on food labels
- have and know how to use measuring cups and spoons
- measure and record blood glucose levels

In addition, advanced carbohydrate counting requires

- assessment that the person has mastered basic carbohydrate counting and is able and willing to progress
- the use of an insulin or medication regimen that matches well with advanced carbohydrate counting
- the ability to use an individualized insulin:carbohydrate ratio and sensitivity factor

- the ability and willingness to check and record blood glucose before meals and at bedtime (at least 4 times per day)
- the ability to safely carry insulin and other supplies

EDUCATOR SKILLS AND TIME

In teaching carbohydrate counting, be mindful of the "process of diabetes medical nutrition therapy" (12), the four-step model that consists of

- assessment of the person's metabolic, nutrition, and lifestyle parameters
- identification and negotiation of nutrition goals
- intervention designed to achieve individualized goals
- evaluation of knowledge, application of intervention, and clinical and behavioral outcomes

This model is a cyclical and continuous process that fosters self-management of diabetes and quality outcomes. The dietitian diabetes educator (RD, CDE) is the health care professional most likely to possess the expertise to teach carbohydrate counting (13), but this book will assist other health care professionals with sufficient knowledge of diabetes to teach this meal planning approach as well.

Teaching basic carbohydrate counting requires at least two one-hour visits over several weeks or months. The visits must sufficiently allow you to evaluate the person's knowledge and application. You can teach the basics of carbohydrate counting during individual counseling or in a group setting with several participants. Clearly, the group setting is more cost-effective.

At least two one-hour sessions are needed for the person to master the concepts of advanced carbohydrate counting and for you to assess the adequacy of knowledge and application of principles. The concepts of advanced carbohydrate counting can be taught in a group setting or individually. However, because fewer people will be taught advanced carbohydrate counting, you are unlikely to have a sufficient number of people to warrant group education.

To maximize efficiency, speed the learning process, and help the person with diabetes achieve glycemic control as quickly as possible, consider taking advantage of communication technologies rather than always providing service in person. Ask your patients to fax or e-mail records that include blood glucose values, food, and medication in advance of teaching sessions. Encourage patients to utilize data management systems available with many glucose meters and insulin pumps. Follow up teaching sessions with phone calls or emails.

HELPFUL CARBOHYDRATE COUNTING TEACHING TOOLS

- Measuring equipment (see list of measuring equipment on pages 11–12) to teach portion size and the importance of portion size control
- Food packages with Nutrition Facts of commonly purchased food items and convenience foods to demonstrate use of carbohydrate information
- Calculator
- Foods and/or food models for educator to demonstrate and/or people to use to identify proper portions (one resource is Nasco: 800-558-9595 or *www.eNasco.com*)
- Handouts: Appendix 2: How Much Carbohydrate to Eat and When?; Appendix 3: Carbohydrate Counting Resources; "Handy Hand Guide," page 12
- Restaurant menus and fast food and restaurant resources that provide carbohydrate counts
- Record keeping form (see Appendix 4 for an example)
- Various insulin syringes, pens, injection aids, and insulin pumps

CHAPTER TWO

Basic Carbohydrate Counting

THE NUTS AND BOLTS

Each concept taught in basic carbohydrate counting builds on the previous one to provide the scope of knowledge and skills a person needs. Appendix 5 is a teaching checklist.

Why count carbohydrate? People need a reason to be motivated to make changes. Provide an understanding of the rationale for counting carbohydrate: "Carbohydrate is the main nutrient that raises blood glucose levels. It raises blood glucose the most and the quickest after meals. Protein and fat raise blood glucose levels minimally. Focusing on the nutrient that most impacts blood glucose levels can help you achieve blood glucose control. All foods containing carbohydrate raise blood glucose to about the same degree in about the same amount of time."

Foods that contain carbohydrate. Don't assume that people know which foods contain carbohydrate. Commonly, people believe that the only foods that contain carbohydrate are starches—cereals, bread, pasta and starchy vegetables—and do not realize that fruit, milk, or sugary foods also contain carbohydrate. To assess a person's knowledge, ask "What foods do you think contain carbohydrate?"

Carbohydrate is healthy. Once they realize that carbohydrate raises blood glucose levels, some people react by eating less carbohydrate than they need. The promise of weight loss promoted by low-carbohydrate, high-protein diets also

Foods that Contain Carbohydrate

Breads, cereals, pasta, and grains

Rice, beans, and starchy vegetables: potatoes, corn, peas

Fruit and fruit juices

Milk and yogurt (most cheeses contain minimal carbohydrate)

Sugary foods: regular soda, fruit drinks, jelly beans, gum drops

Sweets: cake, cookies, chocolate candy

cultivates this belief. Educate people that most carbohydrate-containing foods are among the healthiest to eat—grains, fruits, vegetables, and low- or fat-free milk and yogurt. Carbohydrate-containing foods are also good sources of many essential vitamins and minerals. These are exactly the foods all Americans are encouraged to eat as the foundation of their eating plan. Reinforce the idea that careful attention to the portions of carbohydrate-containing foods is critical to blood glucose control.

Sweets. The ADA recommends teaching people how to work sucrose and sucrose-containing foods into the meal plan as carbohydrate. This recommendation is based on evidence that including sucrose in the meal plan does not impair blood glucose control; rather, it is the total amount of carbohydrate consumed versus carbohydrate type that impacts blood glucose levels (4). With this science in hand, teach people that they can eat sweets safely on occasion but to eat them in moderation due not only to the amount of sugar and calories, but also because sweets typically contain varying amounts of fat, saturated fat, and cholesterol. Provide people with tips for eating fewer and smaller portions of sweets, e.g., share dessert in a restaurant, ask for child-size or small portions at an ice cream shop or fast food restaurant, keep large portions of sweets out of the house.

A carbohydrate serving. People need to have a sense of how much food represents one, two, three, or more servings of carbohydrate. They need to be able to translate the amount of carbohydrate they should eat into real amounts of food.

In the language of diabetes exchanges, one serving of a starch, fruit, or milk equals about 15 grams of carbohydrate. The fact that 15 grams equals one serving is a helpful concept to teach. This is because the diabetes exchange servings may be familiar to people with diabetes and the servings that represent about 15 grams of carbohydrate are reasonable portions of most foods (although some 15-gram portions are quite small, i.e., 1/3 cup rice). However, recognize that some people, especially those new to diabetes, might not understand or have experience with the concept that carbohydrate serving equals 15 grams of carbohydrate.

Also, people can get confused between a "diabetes serving" and a "food label serving." Teach that many times they are the same, but in many instances they are different.

Food	Diabetes Serving	(Carbohydrate grams)*	Food Label Serving	(Carbohydrate grams)*
SAME				
Milk	1 cup/8 oz	(12)	1 cup/8 oz	(12)
Bread	1 slice/1 oz	(15)	1 slice/1 oz	(15)
DIFFERENT				
Fruit juice	1/2 cup/4 oz	(15)	1 cup/8 oz	(30)
Hot cereal	1/2 cup, prepared	(15)	1 cup, prepared	(30)

*Approximate values based on *Exchange Lists for Meal Planning*.

In addition, point out that the gram amount listed after serving size in the Nutrition Facts refers to the weight of the item, not the carbohydrate content; for carbohydrate counting, the person needs to use the grams given as total carbohydrate.

Table 1 shows the categories of foods that contain carbohydrate, protein, and fat. Use this chart to point out the different macronutrients in foods and the amount of food equal to 15 grams of carbohydrate or one serving of common foods.

Amount of total daily carbohydrate. The need for carbohydrate relates to calorie needs. Calorie and carbohydrate needs depend on height, weight and weight history, usual food habits and daily schedule, level of physical activity, blood glucose control, and blood lipid levels. According to ADA nutrition recom-

TABLE 1: Nutrients				
Food Group	Serving*	Carbohydrate (g) 4 calories per gram	Protein (g) 4 calories per gram	Fat (g) 9 calories per gram
Bread	1 slice	15	3	0
Cereal, dry	1 oz	15	3	†
Cereal, cooked	1/2 cup	15	3	†
Pasta	1/2 cup	15	3	†
Starchy vegetable	1/3 to 1/2 cup	15	3	0
Fruit, fresh	1 medium piece	15	0	0
Fruit juice	1/3 to 1/2 cup	15	0	0
Fruit, canned, no sugar added	1/2 cup	15	0	0
Vegetable	1/2 cup cooked	5	0	0
Vegetable	1 cup raw	5	0	0
Milk, fat free	1 cup	12	8	0
Yogurt, plain, nonfat	3/4 cup	12	8	0
Sugary foods	1 serving	varies	varies	varies
Sweets	1 serving	varies	varies	varies
Meats	3 oz cooked	0	21	varies
Fats— margarine, mayonnaise, oil	1 tsp	0	0	5

Alcohol contains 7 calories per gram and is considered a nutrient.
*Servings are according to servings in *Exchange Lists for Meal Planning.*
† Depends on the cereal.

mendations, the percentage of calories a person should eat as carbohydrate varies and should be individualized based on the above factors (4). Generally, Americans eat about 40–50% of their calories as carbohydrate. People who tend to eat more "meat and potatoes" might eat closer to 40% of their calories as carbohydrate, whereas people who eat small portions of protein or are vegetarian might eat 50% or more of their calories as carbohydrate.

Appendix 6 provides general guidelines, based on eating 45–50% of calories as carbohydrate, for determining the number of calories and amount of carbohydrate people need. This table also provides the number of servings to suggest from the food groups that contain carbohydrate. For many average-sized adults, a reasonable starting point is about 60–75 grams or 4–5 servings of carbohydrate per meal.

Distributing carbohydrate into meals and snacks. The number of meals and snacks a person eats should be based on two factors.

- Current food habits and daily schedule: Understanding a person's food habits and general daily schedule casts light on blood glucose results and control. Learn how and why they divide their food between meals and snacks. Find out whether they eat three meals a day, snack throughout the day, or eat three meals and an evening snack. Perhaps they skimp on breakfast and eat a large dinner, which could explain why postdinner blood glucose levels are the highest of the day. If they include snacks, find out why. Are they using snacks to cover their insulin dose to prevent hypoglycemia?
- Types and doses of medications: Consider this information in light of their food intake and eating schedule. How well is this routine controlling blood glucose levels? Do food habits, daily schedule, and diabetes medications work in sync? If they are at odds, the medication regimen should be adjusted first. It's easier for someone to change medication than to change lifelong food habits.

After exploring and considering the above factors, divide the amount of carbohydrate into meals and possibly one or more snacks. Strive for a similar amount of carbohydrate at meals and snacks throughout the day and from day to day. Recognize that the average American eats a light breakfast, a slightly heavier lunch, and the biggest meal at dinner.

The decision to include planned snacks, and when to eat them, is based on achieving a balance between food habits and preferences and prevention of hypoglycemia (if they take a medication that can cause hypoglycemia). If someone doesn't want to include snacks and either takes no medication or one without risk of hypoglycemia, then snacks are unnecessary. Snacks are also unnecessary for someone who uses rapid- or short-acting insulin as MDI or in CSII. A young child with a small appetite at meals or difficult-to-control nighttime hypoglycemia might need one or more snacks a day, as would an athletic adult or someone with long intervals between meals. Bedtime snacks are occasionally needed based on activity earlier in the day and bedtime glucose level.

Appendix 2 provides a sample handout to help people learn how much carbohydrate to eat, how to divide the carbohydrate into meals and snacks, and an option to provide two sample meals.

Servings versus grams. Should you teach people to count grams of carbohydrate or servings of carbohydrate? Some educators believe that, if someone is familiar with the diabetic exchange system, the person knows that 15 grams of carbohydrate is a serving or "choice." People who prefer the choice method can divide 15 into the total grams of carbohydrate given on the label. The downside of only teaching servings is that people have no basis for relating the Nutrition Facts on labels or other resources that provide gram counts to grams of carbohydrate. Some educators believe that teaching people to count grams of carbohydrate is more precise and makes it easier to use various resources. In reality, providing both is helpful to people doing basic carbohydrate counting. People who learn advanced carbohydrate counting will need the precision that comes with counting grams of carbohydrate.

Portion control. People often believe that "healthy eating" is simply a matter of choosing and eating healthy foods. That's just one part of the equation. People must also learn that portion size matters. It is now common for the portions of many supermarket and restaurant foods to be oversized, making it difficult for people to understand what the educator is defining as a portion. Apples are a healthy choice, but the average apple in the supermarket is 1 1/2–2 carbohydrate servings (6–8 oz) and contains about 23–30 grams of carbohydrate. Give people practical opportunities to learn proper portion sizes.

- Use food models that demonstrate portion sizes
- Ask people to use measuring tools to produce the correct portions of dry cereals, nuts, or raisins
- Convey how many ounces 1 or 2 servings of fresh fruit should be and encourage them to weigh fresh fruits in the supermarket produce aisle
- Practice using the Nutrition Facts from food labels

People need these common measuring tools:

- Measuring cups for liquids and solids
- Measuring spoons

- Food scale: Encourage people to purchase an inexpensive scale ($5–10) to measure foods that don't have food labels, e.g., fresh fruit, fresh vegetables, bagels, meat. More expensive food scales are available, such as scales that provide the gram weight and grams of carbohydrate ($120–200).
- Nutrition Facts on labels: This is one of the best sources to define a serving as well as one of the best sources for the grams of carbohydrate. Encourage people to read the Nutrition Facts on products. Make sure they realize that the nutrition information provided is for one serving. Reinforce that one food label serving may not be equal to an exchange serving.
- Eyes: Help people train their eyes to judge portions—no special equipment is needed as people become more skilled at judging portion sizes.

Because it is unlikely that most people will continuously weigh and measure their foods, suggest that they:

- Use similar bowls, plates, and cups. For example, if they drink milk, encourage them to use a measuring cup a few times to learn what 8 oz (1 serving) of milk is, then pour it into a glass they regularly use and make a mental note of the spot on the glass 8 ounces of milk comes up to.
- Weigh and measure foods once a week to keep the eyes in check.
- Use the scales in the produce aisle to check weights of fresh fruit and vegetables.

Some educators find it helpful to teach the "handy hand guides" to help people eat foods in proper portions when they cannot, or prefer not to, measure. Point out that a large male may have a "two-cup" fist.

Hand Guide	Example
Thumb tip = 1 tsp	1 serving of mayonnaise or salad dressing
Thumb = 1 oz	1 serving cheese or peanut butter
Palm = 3 oz	1 serving cooked meat (boneless)
Tight fist = 1/2 cup	1 serving frozen yogurt
Loose fist or handful = 1 cup	1 serving vegetables or pasta

Provide resources for carbohydrate counts. If people are familiar with and have the *Exchange Lists for Meal Planning* or another meal planning tool with the carbohydrate count of common foods, ask them to use it. This amount of information is sufficient for people who do basic carbohydrate counting and do not eat a wide variety of foods. Most people need additional carbohydrate counting resources and need to learn how to use them (Appendix 3). Provide guidance about what resources would be most helpful based on their eating habits. If they like to eat at fast food restaurants, advise people to get the carbohydrate counts published by or on the web sites of restaurants they frequent. If they primarily cook from scratch, then a book or web site with carbohydrate counts for fresh and unprocessed foods, such as *Bowes and Church Food Values of Portions Commonly Used,* will help.

Nearly all packaged, canned, and prepared foods have Nutrition Facts on the label. In general, the foods without Nutrition Facts are fresh fruits, vegetables, and other fresh produce, and fresh meat, poultry, and seafood. The total carbohydrate count is required on nearly all foods that have a label. Important details to teach about the food label:

- The Nutrition Facts are for one serving of the food. The person needs to take note of the serving and consider the portion they will eat to correctly figure how much carbohydrate they will eat. Serving sizes on food labels are uniform and defined by the FDA. For example, 1 serving of bread weighs 30 grams (or 1 oz) but contains 15 grams of carbohydrate. One serving of juice is 8 ounces by fluid volume but contains approximately 30 grams of carbohydrate. Servings must be noted in grams as well as household measures, e.g., 1 slice, 10 crackers, or 8 ounces.
- Food label serving sizes are not necessarily the same as exchange serving sizes (see above on page 8).
- The total carbohydrate count includes all the components under total carbohydrate, dietary fiber, sugars, and sugar alcohols (when included).
- There is no need to pay special attention to sugars. They are counted as part of total carbohydrate. "Sugars" are defined by FDA as both naturally occurring sugars and added sugars or all mono- and disaccharides.
- Some foods labeled "sugar free" or "no added sugar" contain sugar alcohols (polyols), which average 2 calories per gram. Grams of polyols appear on the Nutrition Facts as a subcategory of total carbohydrate. For carbohydrate counting (15), if:

- total carbohydrate in the food comes from polyols, and there are less than 10 grams per serving, the carbohydrates do not need to be counted if three or less servings are eaten per day
- total carbohydrate in the food comes from polyols, and there are more than 10 grams per serving, divide total carbohydrate in half then count it
- polyols are just one source of carbohydrate, divide grams of polyols in half and subtract that amount from total carbohydrate for counting
- The nutrition claims "sugar free," "reduced sugars," "no added sugar," and "no sugar added" do not mean the food is carbohydrate or calorie free. People still need to look at the amount of total carbohydrate and count it.

Protein and fat. These nutrients have far less impact on blood glucose levels than carbohydrate. Read more about protein and fat under Special Considerations on page 42. Though the impact of protein and fat on glycemia is minimal, their impact on nutrient intake and calories is clearly important. Communicate this point and provide people with general guidelines about protein and fat.

Protein
- Eat two or three 3-ounce servings of cooked meat or meat substitute per day. This amount might not be sufficient protein for children, pregnant or lactating women, athletes, or larger-than-average–size adults.
- Encourage consumption of protein foods that are lean and lower in saturated fat and cholesterol.
- Encourage low-fat preparation methods for protein foods.

Fat
- Define a serving of fat: 5 grams of fat = one serving
- Teach the number of fat servings that is appropriate for each individual. Refer to Appendix 6: How Much Carbohydrate? to determine the appropriate amount of fat for various calorie ranges.
- If the person eats too much fat and is overweight, provide general information about what foods contain fat and ways to cut down on fat.
- The ADA recommends that ≤10% of total daily calories come from saturated fats (4), so provide people with ways to reduce saturated fat intake, such as using fat-free milk and reduced-fat cheese and eating smaller and fewer portions of protein.

CASE STUDIES

Mary

Situation: Mary is a 52-year-old married woman who has had type 2 diabetes for 4 years. She works 3 days/week, about 8:30 a.m. to 5:00 p.m., as an office receptionist. Mary's family physician referred her to the diabetes education program at the hospital. Mary wants to lose about 20 pounds.

Data: Ht: 5'4"; Wt: 164 lb, weight stable within 3 pounds for 8 years; HbA1c range: 7.8–to 8.6% over the last 2 years

Diabetes medications: Before breakfast: 850 mg Glucophage, 4 mg Amaryl; before dinner: 850 mg Glucophage

Food habits/daily schedule: Work days: Wakes: 7 a.m.; Med: 7:30 a.m.;

Breakfast: 7:30 a.m.: 4 oz orange juice, 1 1/2 cups Cornflakes, 1 cup 2% milk, 1 small banana, coffee with 2% milk and sugar substitute

Lunch: 12:30 p.m.: 6" sub sandwich (ham and cheese or turkey and cheese), 1 1/2-oz bag pretzels, 1 large apple or orange (from home), diet soda

Midafternoon snack: 3:00 p.m.: 1 package (6) peanut butter crackers, diet soda

Dinner: 6:30 p.m.: Tossed salad with 2 Tbsp regular dressing, 1 cup green or yellow vegetable, 1–1 1/2 cups rice, potatoes, or pasta, 4 oz cooked beef, chicken, or fish.

Bedtime snack: 9:30 p.m.: Either 1 cup light ice cream or frozen yogurt or 6 oz fruited yogurt

Nonwork days during week: Gets up, takes meds, and eats breakfast an hour later than on work days. Eats a similar breakfast; lunch is frozen light entrée with piece of fruit; and snacks and dinner are similar.

Weekends: Schedule is similar to nonwork days. Eats one or two dinners out at Chinese, Italian, or Japanese restaurants. Might have glass of wine at meal and split a dessert.

Physical activity: Moves around at work. On nonwork days, tries to do a 20-minute walk. Weekends does gardening and housework.

SMBG: Checks 1–2 times/day, fasting and before dinner. Average fasting: 160–220 mg/dl; average predinner: 200–240 mg/dl.

Meal planning: The only diabetes education Mary has had is one session with a dietitian at the hospital. She was provided with a 1500 calorie meal plan and a booklet with diabetes exchanges. She attempts to follow it, but doesn't understand it too well and doesn't feel that all the foods she eats are included. She wants to know how to fit a wider variety of foods into her diet, including convenience and restaurant foods.

Action plan:
1. Have Mary attend a class on type 2 diabetes management. This will help her learn the essentials of diabetes management and the importance of blood glucose control as well as the basics of carbohydrate counting. Reinforce that eating a similar amount of carbohydrate at meals and snacks each day will help control blood glucose.
2. Provide guidelines about how much carbohydrate to eat and when. Provide this in servings (15 grams of carbohydrate/serving), because she is familiar with the *Exchange Lists for Meal Planning*, and in grams, so she can begin to interpret the Nutrition Facts labels. Work with Mary to create two sets of sample meals using both the carbohydrate servings and grams (Appendix 2).
3. Provide Mary with a list of suggestions to help her trim calories.
4. Ask if Mary is willing to increase the frequency of her blood glucose monitoring to 2–3 times/day. Encourage her to vary the times that she checks blood glucose to include fasting, premeal, and 2-hour postprandial checks to see the effect of carbohydrate on her blood glucose.

Mary's goals:
1. Use food measuring tools when eating at home to become more familiar with servings of foods. Weigh fruits in supermarket to determine size and buy smaller if appropriate.
2. Attempt to plan and eat meals according to how much carbohydrate is suggested.
3. Check blood glucose 2–3 times/day and record. Fax records that include blood glucose, carbohydrate intake, and activity in two weeks and bring them to the visit in one month.
4. Gather the Nutrition Facts labels from foods she regularly eats and ones she wants to learn how to include.
5. Collect the take-out menus from her four favorite restaurants.

Follow-up:
By telephone two weeks later, after educator received faxed blood glucose records:

1. Mary's fasting blood glucose has not improved, but predinner blood glucose has improved. Results of PPGs range from 170 to 245.

2. By measuring foods, Mary has observed that she has been eating more than she needs.

Individual counseling one month later:

1. Review Mary's use of carbohydrate counting and the amount of food she is eating.
2. Review blood glucose records. Weigh and assess change in weight.
3. Using food labels, have Mary figure the number of servings in the portion size of the food she eats.
4. Using restaurant menus, discuss Mary's current choices, suggest healthier choices, and discuss strategies to decrease restaurant portions.
5. Determine Mary's need for additional carbohydrate counting resources.
6. Note that you will contact her physician to recommend an increased Glucophage and/or Amaryl dose to further help lower her fasting blood glucose levels.

Dave

Situation: Dave is a 69-year-old widower who has had type 2 diabetes for 16 years. He is a retired mechanical engineer who does volunteer work at local schools and other community programs. He has a "lady friend" whom he sees several times a week. She might prepare dinner for Dave or they eat out. Dave is frustrated with his swings in blood glucose levels. He requested that his nurse practitioner refer him to a dietitian diabetes educator in the community who, according to his diabetes support group friends, teaches carbohydrate counting.

Data: Ht: 5'10"; Wt: 198 lb, weight has increased slowly since retirement; HbA1c range: 8.7%, up from a usual 7.3–7.6% over the last three years.

Diabetes medications: Before breakfast: 45 mg Actos, 9 U regular insulin; before lunch: 9 U regular insulin; before dinner: 9 U regular insulin; before bed: 18 U NPH insulin

Food habits/daily schedule: Week days: Wakes: 8 a.m.; Med: 8:15 a.m.;

Breakfast: 8:30 a.m.: 8 oz orange juice, 2 packages instant oatmeal, 1 Tbsp raisins, 1/2 cup 1% milk; or 8 oz orange juice, 2 cup mixture of Cheerios, Spoonsize Shredded Wheat, and All Bran with Fiber, 1 cup 1% milk, 1 slice whole-wheat bread with butter. One morning a week: Fast food sausage and egg on biscuit or 2 donuts.

Lunch: 12:30–1:30 p.m.: Packs 2 sandwiches with ham or turkey and cheese, small bag of chips, and large apple or banana, or has a fast food hamburger or fried chicken sandwich with medium French fries and iced tea or diet soda.

Dinner: 6:30 –7:30 p.m.: Ranges from frozen entrée with protein, starch, and vegetable with dinner roll and salad; to balanced meal made by "lady friend"— meat, starch, vegetable, salad with 8–10 oz wine; to dinner out at an Italian, Mexican, Chinese, or American restaurant. Might split a dessert once or twice a week.

Bedtime snack: 10:00–11:00 p.m.: 6 sugar-free sandwich cookies or 1 cup sugar-free light ice cream.

Weekends: Schedule is similar to weekdays.

Physical activity: Moves around when he volunteers at the school. In good weather he takes a 20-minute walk in his neighborhood. Some gardening once or twice a week in good weather.

SMBG: Was advised recently to check more often; had only been doing first thing in the morning (fasting). Now checking about 3 times a day both before and after some meals. Average fasting: 140–180 mg/dl; average prelunch: 60–90 mg/dl (some feelings of hypoglycemia when below 80); average 2-h postdinner: 220–260 mg/dl.

Meal planning: Dave's wife was alive when he was diagnosed with diabetes. They received a meal plan for 1800 calories and attended a series of classes about type 2 diabetes. His wife attended to his meal plan before she became ill. Dave then took the attitude that he would try to eat healthy as much as possible and eat 3 meals a day at about the same time. That was as much as he felt he could do, especially during his wife's long illness. Dave's knowledge of carbohydrates and servings is minimal. The dietitian believes that Dave has the ability to learn basic carbohydrate counting and just needs to learn how to assess the impact of the amount of carbohydrate he eats on his blood glucose levels.

Action plan:
1. Teach Dave the skills of basic carbohydrate counting. Encourage him to purchase a book with carbohydrate counts for basic and convenience foods as well as one for fast foods.
2. Encourage Dave to begin weighing and measuring foods when eating at home and to learn the "handy guides" to estimate portions when he's not able to measure foods. Review healthy choices in fast food restaurants. Using Appendix 6, provide Dave with a range of carbohydrate to eat at meals.

3. Suggest that Dave would improve his glucose control by losing a few pounds. Agree on a reasonable goal weight. However, as he strives to intensify his blood glucose control, he may need more insulin and is likely to better utilize the calories he eats, which usually results in weight gain. Advise him to trim the amount of fat he eats as well as to observe proper portion sizes. As he controls portion sizes and loses weight, he may then need less insulin.
4. Provide Dave with record-keeping forms (Appendix 4) to keep food, carbohydrate counts, and blood glucose.

Dave's goals:

1. Purchase carbohydrate counting guides via an online book store.
2. Weigh and measure foods when he eats dinner at home and at his "lady friend's."
3. Check blood glucose levels 3–4 times a day, rotating between before and after meals.
4. Keep food, carbohydrate, and blood glucose records for 2 weeks and fax them in. Schedule a phone conversation for 2 weeks and a follow-up appointment for one month.

Follow-up:

By telephone two weeks later, after educator received faxed blood glucose records:

1. All of Dave's blood glucose levels are down about 10–20 mg/dl. He has had an increase in the frequency of mild hypoglycemia before lunch and before bed.
2. The dietitian notes that she will contact Dave's nurse practitioner and suggest that Dave might do better on one injection of insulin glargine (Lantus) at bedtime (see action curves on pages 23–25) and rapid-acting insulin before meals, believing this will diminish the hypoglycemia as his glycemic control improves.
3. By reading books and food labels, Dave has observed that he had been in the habit of overeating. He has lost a pound by decreasing the amount of fat he eats.

Individual counseling one month later:

1. Dave's nurse practitioner agreed to work with Dave to change his insulin regimen, and Dave will visit the nurse practitioner when he is

ready to do so. The nurse practitioner agreed to have Dave use his new insulin regimen in combination with advanced carbohydrate counting when the dietitian assessed he was able to do so. The dietitian explained that this meal planning approach was likely to help Dave achieve better glucose control and greater flexibility in his food choices and amount of food he needs to eat at meals.

2. Dave's records were complete and showed that he was checking his blood glucose about 3 times a day. The dietitian asked whether Dave would be willing to do more frequent checks when he begins his new insulin regimen.

3. Dave's records showed that he was doing a good job of approximating the amount of carbohydrate he was eating but was still eating more than he needed. Also, he had not made many changes in his fast food or other restaurant choices.

4. Dave decided that he wanted more time before venturing into advanced carbohydrate counting. He will continue to try to eat similar amounts of carbohydrate at meals and keep his records. (See continuation of Dave's case study on page 32 in Advanced Carbohydrate Counting.)

CHAPTER THREE

Advanced Carbohydrate Counting

THE NUTS AND BOLTS

Before teaching a person advanced carbohydrate counting, determine their mastery of all the elements of basic carbohydrate counting with the checklist in Appendix 4. Advanced carbohydrate counting is appropriate for those on MDI or CSII. The special aspects of advanced carbohydrate counting for those using insulin pumps are discussed in a section beginning on page 37.

Understanding insulin action. A person who uses MDI or CSII must know the action, peak, and duration of the insulins they take (Table 2).

Insulin regimens. Twenty-four-hour insulin coverage can be provided with MDI or CSII. CSII uses rapid- or short-acting insulin only. MDI consists of an intermediate- or a long-acting basal insulin and a rapid- or short-acting bolus insulin (Table 3). Premixed insulin combinations, such as 70/30 (a mix of 70% NPH and 30% regular) and 75/25 (a mix of 75% NPH and 25% Humalog), are not useful for people who adjust their insulin doses for carbohydrate counting.

Basal insulin. For MDI, the longer-acting insulin covers the natural release of glucose from the liver and maintains normoglycemia between meals and during sleep. Basal insulin constitutes about 50% of the total daily dose (but can range from 45% to 60%), either given once or split into two doses. Pumps release rapid- or short-acting insulin continuously in very small doses to create basal (background) insulin.

TABLE 2: The Action of Insulins

Insulin	Onset	Peak	Duration
Rapid acting			
lispro (Humalog)	<15 minutes	0.5–1.5 hours	2–4 hours
aspart (Novolog)	<15 minutes	0.5–1.0 hour	1–3 hours
Short acting			
regular	0.5–1 hour	2–3 hours	3–6 hours
Intermediate			
NPH	2–4 hours	4–10 hours	10–16 hours
lente	3–4 hours	4–12 hours	12–18 hours
Long acting			
ultralente	6–10 hours	10–16 hours	18–20 hours
glargine (Lantus)	2–4 hours	peakless	24 hours

Bolus insulin. In either MDI or CSII, rapid- or short-acting bolus insulin is taken to cover the carbohydrate in food. A specific amount of insulin is delivered before or during the meal to match the amount of carbohydrate consumed. The amount is based on the individual's insulin:carbohydrate ratio (see below). Because of the convenience of injecting as the meal begins or once the amount of carbohydrate eaten is known, rapid-acting insulin is most com-

TABLE 3: Common MDI Regimens

Before breakfast	Before lunch	Before evening meal	At bedtime	See Figure
Rapid/Short	Rapid/Short	Rapid/Short	Glargine	1
NPH + Rapid/Short	Rapid/Short	Rapid/Short	NPH	2
NPH + Rapid/Short	—	Rapid/Short	NPH	3
NPH + Rapid/Short	—	NPH + Rapid/Short	—	4
Ultralente + Rapid/Short	Rapid/Short	Rapid/Short	—	5

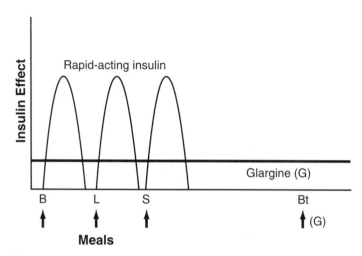

FIGURE 1. Rapid-acting insulin with meals and long-acting insulin at bedtime. **B**, breakfast; **L**, lunch; **S**, supper; **Bt**, bedtime.

monly used as the bolus insulin. Bolus insulin constitutes about 50% of the total daily insulin dose but can range from 40% to 55%.

Insulin delivery vehicles. It's important to discuss options and provide guidelines for insulin delivery that make it comfortable and convenient for the person.

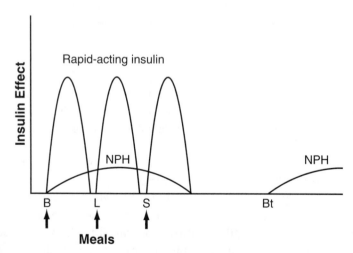

FIGURE 2. Rapid-acting insulin with meals and NPH insulin with breakfast and at bedtime. **B**, breakfast; **L**, lunch; **S**, supper; **Bt**, bedtime.

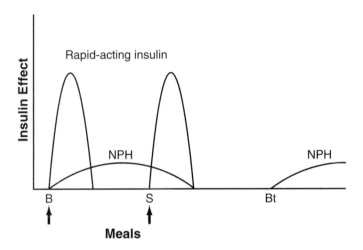

FIGURE 3. Rapid-acting insulin with breakfast and supper and NPH insulin with breakfast and at bedtime. **B**, breakfast; **L**, lunch; **S**, supper; **Bt**, bedtime.

Plastic disposable insulin syringes vary in their volume capacity and needle gauge and length. Syringes are available in 1/3-, 1/2-, and 1-cc capacity; for less than 30 units, a 1/3-cc syringe is best. Needle lengths vary from 5/16" to 1/2" and are available in 28-, 29-, and 30-gauge widths. The higher the gauge number, the thinner the needle and the greater the comfort.

Insulin pens provide added convenience and are available with different needle lengths and gauges. Insulin pens are the size of a thick marking pen and are used with disposable pen needles, ranging in length from 5/16" to 1/2". Pen needle gauge sizes range from 29 to 31. The pens are available as both refillable with disposable insulin cartridges or as completely disposable units with self-contained cartridges. Pens hold up to 315 units of insulin. The advantages of pen therapy include dial or click unit dosing that assures greater accuracy and convenience.

An insulin pump provides the greatest amount of flexibility for insulin dosing. Much smaller doses can be delivered compared to syringes or pens. Most pumps weigh less than 4 oz and are the size of a beeper and worn continuously on a belt or in a pocket. The pump is connected to the person with thin plastic tubing and an infusion set taped to the skin. It delivers rapid- or short-acting insulin subcutaneously through a small, short needle or catheter. The pump is a computerized device that delivers a programmed background amount of basal insulin. Different amounts of basal insulin can

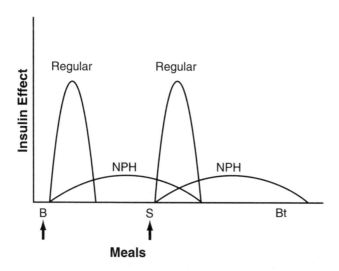

FIGURE 4.   Regular and NPH insulins at breakfast and supper. **B**, breakfast; **L**, lunch; **S**, supper; **Bt**, bedtime.

be programmed to be delivered at various times over 24 hours. The pump wearer presses buttons to allow the pump to deliver bolus doses for food coverage and to correct high blood glucose levels. Pumps can hold up to 315 units of insulin. Proficiency in carbohydrate counting is essential for successful pump therapy (15).

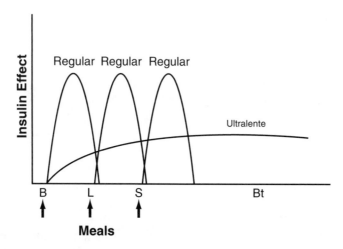

FIGURE 5.   Regular insulin at meals and long-acting insulin at breakfast. **B**, breakfast; **L**, lunch; **S**, supper; **Bt**, bedtime.

Determining insulin needs. The total daily dose (TDD) of insulin can be calculated by a variety of methods. Clinicians often use a calculation of 0.5–1.0 units per kilogram body weight as a starting point and make adjustments based on SMBG results (16). It is optimal to be conservative and make slight incremental increases as results are observed. Slowly titrating up helps prevent hypoglycemia and may assist in determining a person's sensitivity to insulin, which varies from person to person (Table 4). SMBG records are essential in determining the TDD.

Calculating insulin:carbohydrate ratio. The insulin:carbohydrate ratio can be calculated using various methods as detailed below. A person's insulin:carbohydrate ratio will depend on their sensitivity to insulin. Generally, the more sensitive someone is to insulin, the larger the amount of carbohydrate covered by a unit of insulin. Also, because some people are more or less insulin resistant at different times of the day or have different levels of activity during the day, they might need more than one insulin:carbohydrate ratio.

Use whichever method seems most appropriate based on the information at hand. If appropriate, use one method to arrive at an insulin:carbohydrate ratio and then use another method to validate the ratio.

Method #1: Food diary, insulin dose, and SMBG information. Ask the person to keep at least one week of records, including

- fasting, premeal, and PPG SMBG results
- premeal bolus insulin doses

TABLE 4: Insulin Sensitivity

Insulin sensitive	Insulin resistant
Children	Pubescents
Thin people with	Those with type 2 diabetes
type 1 diabetes	Those ill with an infection
Conditioned athletes	Late-term pregnant women
Newly diagnosed with type 1 diabetes	People on steroids

- amount of carbohydrate consumed at meals and other times; it is help-ful for people to eat the same amount of carbohydrate for breakfasts, for lunches, and for dinners for a week

With these records, determine the amount of insulin the person used to cover the carbohydrate con-sumed at each meal by dividing the total grams of carbohydrate by the number of units of insulin (18).

Example
- consumed 72 grams of carbohydrate
- used 5 units of insulin
- 2-hour PPG within target range
- 72 ÷ 5 = 14
- insulin:carbohydrate ratio 1:14

This method is most effective if the person's SMBG records indicate that they are consistently within their PPG targets. If blood glucose is gen-erally not in control and carbo-hydrate intake is varied, this method will be less useful because frequent adjustments will be needed.

The ratios derived by these methods are merely starting points. Some clinicians begin by assuming an insulin:carbohydrate ratio of 1:15 for most adults and a ratio of 1:20 or 1:25 for most children—children tend to be more insulin sensitive. Detailed records of SMBG results, carbohydrate intake, and insulin doses provide useful information to make ratio adjustments. Some people need different ratios for different segments of the day. Remind people to recalculate their insulin:carbohydrate ratio and to use their new ratio if:

- TDD changes more than a cou-ple of units
- Body weight changes more than a couple of pounds
- Lifestyle changes, e.g., exercise, stress, working hours

Method #2: The rule of 500. This rule of thumb, widely used by clinicians to determine the insulin:carbohydrate ratio (18), is based on total (basal + bolus) daily insulin dose (TDD). The TDD is divided into 500. The result is the amount of carbohydrate that one unit of rapid-acting insulin will cover, bringing blood glucose into the target range about 3–4 hours postmeal, or that short-acting insulin will cover in about 5–6 hours postmeal.

Example
- TDD is 36 units
- glucose levels are within target range

- 500 ÷ 36 =13.8 (round up to 14)
- insulin:carbohydrate ratio 1:14

Some clinicians find that dividing 450 (rather than 500) by the TDD is more accurate for short-acting insulin and/or for people who are more insulin resistant (need more insulin to cover carbohydrate).

Method #3: Using the insulin sensitivity factor. Once a person's insulin sensitivity factor (ISF) is calculated (see below), multiplying it by 0.33 provides an insulin:carbohydrate ratio.

Example
- TDD is 25 units
- ISF is 72 mg/dl
- 72 × 0.33 = 23.8 (round up to 24)
- insulin:carbohydrate ratio 1:24

Insulin sensitivity factor. The ISF is defined as the amount of blood glucose (in mg/dl) reduced by 1 unit of rapid- or short-acting insulin. Although different names are used—ISF, correction factor, or supplemental factor—this is the method for calculating the amount of insulin needed to return blood glucose to within the premeal target range.

Two commonly accepted formulas are used as starting points in determining the ISF: the 1500 rule and the 1800 rule. They apply a mathematical constant that expresses the relationship between body size and insulin action. The 1500 rule was developed by endocrinologist Paul C. Davidson, MD. With the introduction of rapid-acting insulin, John Walsh, PA, CDE, a pump specialist (18), modified the 1500 rule into the 1800 rule. Clinicians tend to use the 1800 rule for rapid-acting insulin and/or with insulin-sensitive people and the 1500 rule for short-acting insulin and/or with those who are insulin resistant. Again, these are starting points; trial and error will determine each individual's ISF.

The rules calculate ISF by dividing either 1800 or 1500 by the TDD. No matter which rule is used, recalculate ISF if TDD changes more than a few units.

Examples
- TDD is 34 units
- 1800 ÷ 34 = 52.9 (round up to 53, but it may be easier to round up to 55 or 60)
- ISF is 53 mg/dl: one unit of rapid-acting insulin decreases glucose by 53 mg/dl

- TDD is 34 units
- $1500 \div 34 = 44$
- ISF is 44 mg/dl: one unit of short-acting insulin decreases glucose by 44 mg/dl

Correction or supplemental insulin dose. It is important to identify target blood glucose goals for and with each person. These targets determine the correction doses of insulin by providing a way to measure how much blood glucose is above or below target.

Example
- glucose is 264 mg/dl
- target glucose level is 100 mg/dl
- ISF is 53 mg/dl
- 264 mg/dl −100 mg/dl = 164 mg/dl above target level
- 164 mg/dl ÷ 53 mg/dl = 3.1 units
- the correction dose of insulin is 3 units

Other common methods used to calculate a supplemental insulin dose are:
- One unit of rapid- or short-acting insulin lowers blood glucose 50 mg/dl.
- Providing number of units of rapid- or short-acting insulin per blood glucose ranges (often call a sliding scale), i.e., 100–150 mg/dl: add 1 unit; 151–200 mg/dl, add 2 units.

Premeal insulin dose. To determine the premeal insulin dose, teach people to add the number of units of insulin needed to cover the amount of carbohydrate that will be consumed with the number of units of insulin that will bring the premeal blood glucose back to target. If blood glucose premeal is in the target range, no correction insulin is needed. If premeal blood glucose is below target range, a smaller premeal bolus is needed. See "Correcting hypoglycemia."

Example
- target glucose level is 100 mg/dl
- ISF is 53 mg/dl
- insulin:carbohydrate ratio 1:15
- premeal glucose level is 226 mg/dl
- 60 grams of carbohydrate are to be consumed
- 60 ÷ 15 = 4 units of insulin to cover the carbohydrate
- 226 mg/dl −100 mg/dl = 126 mg/dl

- 126 mg/dl ÷ 53 mg/dl = 2.3 units insulin to decrease the high premeal glucose level
- 4 units + 2.3 units = 6.3 units insulin (insulin pump bolus) or round down to 6 units insulin (if using syringe or pen)

It is important that the high blood glucose that will be brought back to premeal target is actually the premeal blood glucose and not one taken one to two hours after the last meal. A 1- or 2-hour postprandial blood glucose measurement reflects the action of the previous premeal dose of rapid- or short-acting insulin, which is not yet complete. If a postprandial glucose measure is used to calculate a correction dose, there is the possibility of giving too much insulin and causing hypoglycemia. Encourage people to space meals at least 3–4 hours apart and to make sure that the dose they are calculating is based on a true premeal blood glucose.

Pattern management. It's important to review the patterns of blood glucose monitoring results with people. Unexplained and repeated hypo- or hyperglycemia requires modifications in carbohydrate counting calculations, insulin doses, or both. Teach people to check for and note in their records the following:

- Missed meals or snacks
- An amount of carbohydrate consumed that was not factored in to premeal bolus
- Varied eating schedule (if on MDI)
- More or less exercise or activity than usual
- Stress or illness
- Hypoglycemia and treatment used, i.e., amount of carbohydrate
- Other factors that may impact blood glucose levels, e.g., insulin pump infusion set change, alcohol intake

Correcting hyperglycemia. Hyperglycemia can result from inaccurate carbohydrate counting and/or an incorrect premeal insulin dose. Hyperglycemia may also result when insulin action is not timed to accommodate the delayed digestion that occurs with excessive protein or fat intake or gastroparesis. If a person consistently uses a correction dose of insulin, determine why. Use information from SMBG, carbohydrate intake, and insulin doses. Review carbohydrate counts for accuracy. If the calculations are correct, then review the insulin doses. One or more insulin dose changes can be made. Always try one method at a time.

- Decrease the insulin:carbohydrate ratio: use 1 unit of insulin to cover less carbohydrate
- Increase the amount of basal insulin

An increase in physical activity may also help correct hyperglycemia. But it's best to fine-tune insulin doses related to carbohydrate intake first and then incorporate changes for physical activity. Planned exercise time is not always guaranteed to decrease glucose levels. For instance, people with type 1 diabetes may experience hyperglycemia if they exercise while underinsulinized.

Correcting hypoglycemia. Hypoglycemia can result from inaccurate carbohydrate counting, too large an insulin bolus, too much basal insulin, alcohol intake, or unplanned physical activity. Hypoglycemia can also result from taking bolus insulin doses too close together or improperly timing insulin delivery to accommodate gastroparesis or meals with excess protein and/or fat. Review carbohydrate counts for accuracy. If the calculations are correct, then review the insulin doses and timing of insulin action. One or more insulin dose changes can be made. Always try one method at a time.

- Increase the insulin:carbohydrate ratio: use 1 unit of insulin to cover more carbohydrate, e.g., use a ratio of 1:20 instead of 1:15
- Decrease the amount of basal insulin

To correct premeal hypoglycemia, people can be encouraged to take one or more immediate actions:

- Increase the amount of carbohydrate at the meal, but do not increase the premeal insulin dose. Base the amount of additional carbohydrate on the ISF. The person should know the amount of carbohydrate that will raise their blood glucose a certain number of milligrams per deciliter.

Example
- target blood glucose is 100
- premeal blood glucose is 55
- ISF is 35 mg/dl
- insulin:carbohydrate ratio 1:13
- 13 grams of carbohydrate will raise their blood glucose by 35 mg/dl
- he/she needs about 16 grams of carbohydrate to bring glucose to 100 mg/dl or target

This method of treating hypoglycemia is best for people who do not have concerns about their weight. Obviously, eating more adds calories. For those watching calories, reducing insulin is a better approach.

- Decrease the premeal insulin dose using the ISF and insulin:carbohydrate ratio
- Delay the premeal insulin dose until during or the conclusion of the meal to give the food a chance to raise blood glucose level, i.e., check glucose 15–20 minutes after beginning the meal and give insulin with glucose begins to increase

Again, careful SMBG and record keeping will help establish patterns to determine when and how to make adjustments.

Clinicians often use the general rule of 15 to correct hypoglycemia. This rule rests on the belief that 15 grams of carbohydrate raises blood glucose about 50 mg/dl. The person below target range should eat 15 grams of carbohydrate and check blood glucose 15 minutes later; if glucose is not in the target range, the person repeats these actions.

CASE STUDIES
Dave

Situation: About 6 months after learning basic carbohydrate counting, Dave called the dietitian. He noted that his blood glucose levels were still not in control and his recent HbA1c of 8.2% was not much lower than before. His annual retinal exam showed early retinopathy. Dave wants to get more aggressive with his glucose control and learn advanced carbohydrate counting because he plans to live a long time and wants to retain his sight. At their appointment, the dietitian encouraged Dave to first talk with his nurse practitioner to switch to rapid-acting insulin before meals and insulin glargine (Lantus) once a day before bedtime.

Actions:
1. Based on Dave's food records, and using the rule of 500 to double-check, they determined that the insulin:carbohydrate ratio that would work for lunch and dinner was 1:11. They also determined Dave's correction factor based on the 1800 rule. At a TDD of 45 units of insulin, Dave's ISF is about 40 mg/dl.

2. Using his food and blood glucose records, Dave demonstrated his ability to use the formulas to determine how much insulin he would take before meals. He realized this was going to be time-consuming but realized that it made sense.

3. The dietitian cautioned Dave about weight gain. He hadn't made much progress losing weight. She noted it would only get tougher the better his control and the more liberated he felt with his food choices.

4. They set up an appointment for Dave to return in about a month, and Dave agreed to fax his records in two weeks and call with problems or questions.

Stephanie

Situation: Stephanie is a 42-year-old married mother of two teenagers who has had type 1 diabetes for 18 years. Stephanie works full-time with alternating shifts and weekends as a pediatric nurse. Her insulin regimen was changed a month ago from two split, mixed doses of rapid-acting insulin and NPH to insulin glargine (Lantus) at bedtime with premeal rapid-acting insulin. Her nighttime hypoglycemia has decreased, but her daytime SMBG values are erratic, and she struggles to achieve her target premeal glucose level of 120 mg/dl. Stephanie met once with the hospital dietitian for carbohydrate counting. She is returning for a second appointment with one week of SMBG records, insulin doses, and carbohydrate counts.

Data: Ht: 5'6"; Wt: 141 lb; weight gradually increased 6 pounds in past 4 years; HbA1c: 7.8%, 8.2%, and 7.9% in the past year.

Diabetes medication: Uses insulin pen for rapid-acting insulin prebreakfast, prelunch, and predinner according to this sliding scale: if premeal glucose is <100 mg/dl: 3 units; 100–150 mg/dl: 5 units; 151–200 mg/dl: 7 units; 201–250 mg/dl: 10 units; >251 mg/dl: 12 units and check for ketones; bedtime: 9:30 –10:00 p.m. 28 units glargine.

Food habits/daily schedule: Day shift 7:00 a.m. to 3:30 p.m.

Breakfast, 6:00 a.m.: 6 oz orange juice, 1 bowl corn flakes or granola cereal, 8 oz 1% milk, coffee with sugar substitute

Lunch, 11:00 a.m., sometimes delayed until 11:30 a.m.: sandwich from home with 2 slices wheat bread, 2–3 slices turkey or ham and cheese, diet soda; or hospital cafeteria chef salad, 2 Tbsp fat-free dressing, diet soda; or 2 slices cheese pizza and diet soda.

Dinner, 6:00 p.m.: 5 days/week eats at home: Tossed salad with 2 Tbsp fat-free dressing, 1/2 cup green or yellow vegetable, occasional slice of bread, baked chicken or fish, 2–3 small cookies or fruit, sugar-free fruit mix drink or no-sugar-added fruit juice.

Stephanie eats out 2 nights/week at a local pizza shop or Chinese restaurant; no alcohol.

Evening shift 3:00 p.m. to 11:30 p.m.

Breakfast: same, at 9:30 a.m.

Lunch, 2:00 p.m.: leftovers from evening meal or sandwich with piece of fruit, diet soda

Dinner, 7:00 p.m.: at hospital cafeteria: same as day shift lunch.

Snack (on occasion), 9:30 p.m.: apple or banana

Physical activity: Day shift: moderate walking, lifting children, feeding children, and delivering medications. Evening shift: less active.

Days off: 1/2 hour walk, does grocery shopping and housework

SMBG: Checks 4–5 times/day. Average fasting: 90–150 mg/dl; average pre-lunch: 160–250 mg/dl; average predinner: 185–300 mg/dl; average bedtime: 110–190 mg/dl. Uses two different glucose meters, one at home and the hospital floor meter at work. Does not do PPGs.

Action plan:
1. Discuss carbohydrate counts of Stephanie's meals, including restaurant choices.
2. Review SMBG records and sliding scale insulin doses. Point out the differences in the carbohydrate amounts related to specific insulin doses. Review onset, peak, and duration of rapid-acting insulin.
3. Discuss the importance of using one meter to perform SMBG, as adjusting insulin doses based on results from two different meters can cause inconsistencies in calculations. Discuss potential benefit of checking PPG. Develop insulin:carbohydrate ratio and ISF from her records. Use an average of her rapid-acting insulin doses for TDD.
   - Breakfast: 5 units; lunch: 7 units; dinner: 9 units = 21 units lispro + 28 units glargine = 49 units TDD
   - Insulin:carbohydrate ratio: $500 \div 49$ units = 10.2 (round down to 10); use ratio of 1:10
   - ISF: $1800 \div 49 = 36.7$ mg/dl (round up to 37 or 40 mg/dl)
   - Premeal target blood glucose (per physician): 120 mg/dl
4. Discuss when and how to use her formulas. Explain appropriate insulin doses with variations in meals. Ask Stephanie to demonstrate her

ability to apply her insulin:carbohydrate ratio and ISF by planning a variety of typical meals. Note foods and meals that require dosage adjustments based on new insulin doses: 1) eating granola cereal instead of cornflakes results in higher prelunch glucose, 2) predinner glucose numbers are lower when her lunch is a chef salad instead of a sandwich, 3) drinking no-added-sugar fruit juice at dinner resulted in a higher bedtime glucose value than drinking a sugar-free fruit mix beverage, 4) fasting glucose is elevated following evening shift fruit snack at 9:30 p.m., and 5) bedtime and fasting values are elevated following dinner restaurant meals.

5. Ask Stephanie to fax in one week of record, including carbohydrate counts, insulin doses, SMBG values, and any changes in activity levels. Note you will call her after you review the records.
6. Set up follow-up appointment.

Stephanie's goals:
1. Stephanie agreed to carry the meter she uses at home with her to work for SMBG checks to avoid inconsistencies in insulin dose calculations. She did not want to add PPG checks, but agreed to check PPGs twice a day on her days off.
2. Stephanie will use her insulin:carbohydrate ratio and ISF to calculate her premeal doses. She will keep detailed records and fax them in.
3. Stephanie will be more careful assessing the carbohydrate content of restaurant foods and will review the carbohydrate counts on the Nutrition Facts of foods she uses.
4. Stephanie agreed to use measuring equipment at home on occasion to check her portion size.

Follow-up:
1. Stephanie's faxed records showed occasional PPG levels of 180–200 mg/dl range, but most blood glucose values improved to be ±30 mg/dl of her premeal target of 120 mg/dl. Prelunch glucose numbers are more consistent and close to her target.
2. Stephanie learned that, using her insulin:carbohydrate ratio, she had more variety in food choices while she improved her control.
3. Stephanie improved her carbohydrate calculations of restaurant meals by measuring similar foods at home. She had been estimating her rice portion as 1 cup, and she actually consumes 2 cups when having a Chi-

nese meal. She increased her predinner dose accordingly, which resulted in improved bedtime control.

4. After two months of advanced carbohydrate counting, Stephanie's HbA1c decreased to 6.9%. She lost one pound, and noted that she is doing better at estimating carbohydrate counts because she does not usually need supplemental insulin premeal.

CHAPTER FOUR

Advanced Carbohydrate Counting Using an Insulin Pump

THE NUTS AND BOLTS

It's essential that a person learn and use advanced carbohydrate counting for several weeks or months before beginning pump therapy.

Basal rates. Pumps provide flexibility for meal times and fine-tuning insulin doses. The background, or basal rate, of insulin can be set for different amounts at different times of the day, depending on the user's individual needs. Today's pumps can be set for different basal rate programs over the course of 24 hours. Basal rate requirements can differ day-to-day, depending on hormonal changes (i.e., stage of menstrual cycle), physical activity, and work schedules. Ideally, when basal rates are set properly, premeal blood glucose levels do not fluctuate by more than 30 mg/dl. Basal rates that are correctly set permit the pump user to delay or skip meals, have more flexibility with meal choices, and sleep later than their usual wake-up time. It is important to first establish and fine-tune the basal rates in order to determine that the insulin:carbohydrate ratio used for bolus doses is correct.

Bolus doses. The insulin:carbohydrate ratio is used to match bolus insulin to the amount of carbohydrate consumed. Bolus doses can be fine-tuned to deliver insulin according to the pump wearer's needs. A bolus can be given all at once; some pumps can be programmed for bolus delivery in increments over time or split between both normal and extended delivery. Pump users need to learn to combine these ways of delivering their total meal bolus based on information from SMBG, bolus doses, and meal intake records. The addition of a correction dose, if needed, is added to the premeal bolus dose.

37

Extending a bolus to be delivered slowly over several hours provides insulin coverage for those foods or situations that increase the blood glucose gradually:

- a long dinner, such as a buffet, or special holiday dinner
- a cocktail party, or "grazing" situation
- some ethnic meals, including pizza, Italian, Mexican, and Chinese
- high-protein and -fat meals
- high-fiber or low–glycemic index snacks and meals
- gastroparesis
- illness

CASE STUDY
John

Situation: John is a 34-year-old married man who has had type 1 diabetes for 20 years. He has worn an insulin pump for 4 years. He is a high school English teacher and coaches sports teams after school. John's endocrinologist referred him to the diabetes education program for a carbohydrate counting "refresher." In the past year, John's HbA1c values have increased, he is using a lot of insulin correction boluses for frequent higher than target premeal glucose results, and he has lost weight.

Data: Ht: 5'10"; Wt: 163 lb; 5 pound weight loss in the past year, previous weight stable; HbA1c range: 7.6–8.5% in the past year; 6.5–7.2% over the previous 2 years.

Diabetes medication: Rapid-acting insulin via pump.
- average TDD: 42 units, range 38–46 units; basal total: 18.35 units/ 24 hours
- basal rates: midnight–3 a.m.: 0.8 unit/hour; 3:00–7:30 a.m.: 0.9 unit/ hour; 7:30 a.m.–5:30 p.m.: 0.8 unit/hour; 5:30 p.m.–midnight: 0.6 unit/ hour
- average premeal bolus doses: breakfast: 4 units; lunch: 4–8 units; snack: 2 units; dinner 5–7 units; snack 1.5 units
- insulin:carbohydrate ratio 1:15
- ISF: 40 mg/dl
- 2-hour PPG target: 180 mg/dl; premeal target: 100 mg/dl

SMBG: Premeal SMBG 4 time a day. Fasting range: 90–140s mg/dl; prelunch range: 250–280 mg/dl; predinner range: 56–135 mg/dl;bedtime range: 160–200 mg/dl. Notices higher fasting and lower prelunch blood glucose numbers on weekends. Has occasional predinner hypoglycemia (2–3 days/week).

Food habits/daily schedule: Week days: wakes 5:45 a.m.

Breakfast, 6:30 a.m.: 4 oz orange or apple juice, deli shop bagel with 2 Tbsp light cream cheese, 1 small banana, black coffee with sugar substitute

Lunch, 11:30 a.m.: sandwich from home, 2 slices white or rye bread with 3–4 oz chicken, turkey, or ham, or scoop of tuna salad, small bag potato chips or piece of fruit or 6 oz container fat-free yogurt with fruit, diet soda

Midafternoon snack, 3:00 p.m.: large apple or medium banana, small bag pretzels, diet soda

Dinner, 6:15 p.m.: Tossed salad with 2 Tbsp diet dressing, 1/2–1 cup green vegetable, 2 dinner rolls, 1 cup potatoes or rice or 2 cups pasta, 4–5 oz baked chicken, roast beef, fish, or seafood, diet iced tea

Bedtime snack: occasional dish of ice cream or sugar-free pudding and 2–4 cookies

Weekends: Wakes 7:45 a.m. Juice and fried egg sandwich; similar lunch; dinner out every Saturday at local Italian restaurant, pub, or bar & grill, with 2 glasses lite beer; Sunday dinner similar to weekdays.

Physical activity: During school year: light walking in school, runs 1 mile in late afternoons 2–3 days/week; weekends and in summer: runs 1–2 miles in mornings 3 days/week.

Action plan:
1. Review John's SMBG records. Discuss glucose patterns, i.e., reasons why his weekend fasting and weekday prelunch glucose levels run higher and his weekend prelunch glucose levels are lower than on weekdays.
2. Discuss the impact of exercise. Provide John with guidelines to temporarily decrease his basal rate(s) on exercise days or use a different 24-hour basal program.
3. Review carbohydrate gram amounts in portion sizes of some of his favorite foods, including juice, deli bagels, and yogurt.
4. Ask John to measure his breakfast juice portion, read the Nutrition Facts on bagels of similar size to his (deli-style) in the supermarket

frozen food section and the fat-free fruit yogurt he buys. John agreed to learn the carbohydrate amount of the lite beer he drinks on Saturday nights.

5. Recalculate John's insulin:carbohydrate ratio:
   - Average TDD:42 units
   - 500 ÷ 42 = 11.9 (round up to 12)
   - Based on SMBG results and recent HbA1c increases, suggest an insulin:carbohydrate ratio of 1:12 instead of 1:15. Discuss how/why this may help with his glucose excursions.
6. Encourage John to add PPG checks.
7. Fax one week of SMBG, carbohydrate intake, and boluses records for review.
8. Schedule follow-up phone call 2 weeks later.

John's goals:
1. Measure breakfast juice portion; learn carbohydrate grams for deli-sized bagels, fruited yogurt, and lite beer. Improve accuracy of carbohydrate counting for fruits by purchasing pieces of fruit that are medium in size. He and his wife will weigh individual pieces of fruit in supermarket to get a better feel for the proper size.
2. Use a 1:12 insulin:carbohydrate ratio for meal and snack boluses. Keep detailed records of carbohydrate grams consumed, meal and snack boluses, and use of insulin correction dose.
3. Try a temporary 20% basal rate decrease 1 hour before, during, and for 2 hours after his 1- and 2-mile runs. Keep detailed records of his glucose values before and after runs.
4. Add some PPG checks to his SMBG regimen.
5. Fax in records in 2 weeks.

Follow-up:
1. Using measuring cups and his scale at home, John learned his 4-oz breakfast juice portion is really 8 oz. He read the Nutrition Facts on food labels and calculated 60 grams carbohydrate for his deli bagel, not 30 grams, as he had thought. He also learned the carbohydrate content of his yogurt and 12 oz of lite beer. John recalculated his breakfast total carbohydrate: 8 oz juice: 30 grams; deli bagel: 60 grams; small banana: 15 grams; total: 105 grams. His previous calculation had been 60 grams.
2. With a 1:12 insulin:carbohydrate ratio for boluses (instead of 1:15), he showed marked improvements in glucose levels. Initially, many PPG levels were elevated. He increased most of his meal boluses: breakfast

bolus increased from 4 to 8.75 units based on a total of 105 gm of carbohydrate. Fasting range: 80–125 mg/dl; prelunch range: decreased from mid-to-high 200s to 100–140 mg/dl; predinner range: 85–130 mg/dl; bedtime: 128–180 mg/dl. John now used correction boluses less frequently.

3. On exercise days, John tried a temporary 20% decrease in his basal rate 1 hour before, during, and 2 hours after his runs and had less hypoglycemia. He feels more confident, and plans to increase his running time with an additional decrease in his basal rates.

4. John's HbA1c 3 months after making changes decreased to 6.7%. He has no additional weight loss and is pleased with his stable weight.

CHAPTER FIVE

Special Considerations and Situations

High-protein and/or high-fat meals. For many years it was thought that 50% or more of protein consumed was converted into glucose. Newer research indicates that peripheral glucose concentration does not increase after protein ingestion in normal subjects or people with type 2 diabetes. Protein ingestion actually results in a small decrease in PPG in people with type 2 diabetes. In people with type 1 diabetes, protein has little effect on blood glucose response, unless very large portions are eaten (17). Fat has minimal impact on blood glucose.

A high-protein meal or a high-fat meal—or a combination—may delay the rise of blood glucose from the carbohydrate content of the meal. This may be due, in part, to a delay in stomach emptying. If a person is accustomed to eating a 3–4 oz serving of protein and they eat an 8-oz rib eye steak, they might find that 2-hour PPG is not as high as expected, but the 3- to 5-hour PPG is higher than the 2-hour PPG.

Pizza is another food known to delay the rise of blood glucose and to cause a greater rise than expected (19). Blood glucose impact varies from person to person and situation to situation. People need to learn through monitoring what their reaction is and be provided with techniques to manage various situations. Helpful techniques for those doing advanced carbohydrate counting are

- take rapid-acting insulin after, rather than before, the meal
- split the dose of rapid-acting insulin and take half before the meal and half after the meal

Pumps provide several other options. Read about these on pages 37–38.

Adjusting insulin for fiber content. Teach people doing advanced carbohydrate counting how to adjust their rapid- or short-acting insulin for foods and meals with greater than 5 grams of fiber. This is because the grams of fiber from the total carbohydrate count are, for the most part, not digested and are not absorbed as glucose. The following is an example of how to teach this concept:

A high-fiber breakfast:	Carbohydrate (g)	Fiber (g)
1 cup high-fiber flake cereal	32	6
1 slice whole grain bread	12	3
1 cup fat-free milk	12	0
1 1/4 cup strawberries	15	2
Total	71	11

Subtract the 11 grams of fiber from the 71 grams of carbohydrate.
Figure the insulin dose of rapid- or short-acting insulin based on 60 g of carbohydrate.
Based on an insulin:carbohydrate ratio of 1:15, the insulin dose would be 60 ÷ 15 = 4 units of insulin.

Glycemic index. The glycemic index ranks foods based on the impact of a certain amount of the food on glycemic effect compared to either glucose or white bread. The glycemic index for more than 500 carbohydrate-based foods has been ascertained (20). Some foods, such as rice, have a high glycemic index and others, such as legumes, have a low glycemic index. However, different forms and preparations of the food might cause a different glycemic rise. For this reason and a number of other variables, glycemic index for meal planning has not been endorsed by the ADA (4). However, based on experience, people can develop their "personal glycemic index" as they progress with carbohydrate counting and make changes in their medication based on this experience.

Weight gain. The potential for unwanted weight gain has been documented as people improve glycemic control. People in the intensive treatment group of the DCCT gained an average of 10 lb during the first year of the trial (21). Weight gain that accompanies improved glycemic control is attributed to several factors:

- the loss of fewer calories from glycosuria
- normalizing of glycemia promotes rehydration
- greater frequency of hypoglycemia and need to treat it
- use of one or more medications that are known to cause weight gain

It is also thought that people who do carbohydrate counting might ignore the calories from protein and fat and/or might experiment with the inclusion of higher-calorie foods. One or both of these will increase calorie intake and result in weight gain. It is important to warn people who are striving to achieve glycemic control that weight gain is a potential reality. Encourage them to be cognizant of the protein and fat content of their meals and to recognize that, although they can take more insulin or medication to "cover" the glycemic rise from sweets, ingesting more calories than needed results in weight gain (22).

Restaurant meals. Eating out is common and a part of daily life for many. Ascertain how often the person eats out, the types of restaurants the person visits, and their food choices at various restaurants. With this information, you can prioritize how important knowledge about restaurant eating is and individualize teaching based on the types of restaurants the person eats in and the food choices made. The more often someone eats out, the more important this knowledge will be. For example, if the person eats three lunches a week at a fast food hamburger chain and usually order a double cheeseburger, large fries, and diet beverage, you can

- encourage the person to eat fast food meals less often
- discuss healthier food choices at the restaurant
- provide carbohydrate information for that restaurant chain or information about how to access it

Provide general strategies for healthy restaurant eating, such as how to limit fats, how to practice portion control, and how to use the "handy hand guides" (page 12) to judge portions and carbohydrate count.

Encourage people to check their blood glucose more often when they eat restaurant foods. It will help them recognize that

- eating more food raises their blood glucose higher and they may need more insulin to cover the additional food
- when they eat more protein and fat, it delays the rise in blood glucose levels
- the effects of certain foods on their blood glucose level, i.e., Chinese, Mexican, pizza

Appendix 3 lists several resources about restaurant eating that will help people learn strategies for healthy restaurant eating and that provide carbohydrate counts of restaurant foods. Typically, the carbohydrate counts of restaurant foods are available from the larger chain restaurants and on their web sites.

Special food situations. Eating while on vacation, during holidays, and in other people's homes can present challenges. Encourage people to pay attention to portion sizes. Teach people to look for hidden carbohydrates and learn to count them, such as breading in meat, fish, poultry, and vegetable items and combination dishes. Many holiday and religious traditions include sweetened beverages and unfamiliar foods that contain added carbohydrate as well. When in doubt, encourage people to ask questions about particular foods. The Ethnic and Regional Food Practices Series, listed in Appendix 3, might be helpful in working with people of certain ethnic origins or when eating ethnic cuisines.

Any change in routine or schedule can necessitate a change in insulin doses. For increased activity, such as on vacation, a 10–20% or more decrease in basal insulin doses as well as a change in the insulin:carbohydrate ratio may be necessary. Holidays and eating unfamiliar foods at unusual times may require additional changes and correction doses. Encourage people to "learn from the last time," i.e., keep good records and make adjustments based on patterns.

Alcohol. Alcohol does not require insulin for metabolism. Pure alcohol, such as whiskey, gin, rum, or vodka, contains calories but not carbohydrate. Because alcohol tends to lower blood glucose levels, it does not require extra insulin to cover it. Alcohol can interfere with the release of glycogen for up to 24 hours (most noticeable after 8–10 hours), so it's important to teach people to check blood glucose levels frequently. Advise people to always eat when drinking alcohol. A general recommendation is for the person to eat an additional 15 grams of carbohydrate at bedtime to prevent nocturnal hypoglycemia.

Occasionally, alcohol causes an increase in blood glucose due to the carbohydrate in some alcoholic beverages, such as beer and wine, or the carbohydrate from a mixer, such as juice, cola, or tonic water. If alcoholic beverages are consumed with a meal for which the diabetes medications or insulin is insufficient to cover the meal, blood glucose will increase more than just expected due to insufficient insulin. Teach people to review beer and wine labels in stores or at home and to learn the amount of carbohydrate they are consuming by measuring the amount they consume. Light beer, dry wine, and drinks made with noncaloric mixers require no or fewer insulin dose adjustments. When people drink beer, sweet wine, or a cocktail with a fruit juice or mixer, it's important to count the carbohydrate and make adjustments in premeal insulin doses. Caution people to make conservative changes, because there is increased risk for hypoglycemia associated with alcohol. Detailed SMBG and record keeping can provide useful information for making dosage adjustments.

Activity and exercise. Physical activity generally lowers blood glucose levels. Depending on the type, intensity, and duration of the activity, blood glucose can be lowered up to 36 hours after the activity. To prevent activity-induced hypoglycemia

- Decrease the background insulin/basal rate before, during, and/or after activity. Start with a modest decrease, 10–20%, and adjust as necessary
- Increase carbohydrate consumption (record intake of grams)
- Encourage detailed record keeping to establish blood glucose patterns for activity

Encourage people to make adjustments in carbohydrate intake and/or insulin doses based on their experience and their diabetes and nutrition goals. For example, if someone has increased their activity as a means to achieve weight loss, then it is better to reduce medication to prevent hypoglycemia than to increase calorie intake.

Sick day management and stress. Illness and stress can interfere with blood glucose control. Short-term or minor illness, including dental surgery, colds, sore throat, mild infections, nausea, vomiting, diarrhea, and fever, can cause an increase in blood glucose. Stress, though a normal part of life, can also cause erratic glucose control. Inadequate sleep, too much food, inactivity, and the release of counterregulatory hormones can increase blood glucose. People with type 1 diabetes should check for ketones when blood glucose is 240 mg/dl or higher.

Eating during minor illness may be difficult. Provide guidelines to people so they know who to contact and what to do for specific situations. In general,

- Increase SMBG to detect and treat problems early on.
- Start noncaloric fluids 1–2 hours after any vomiting. Drink the fluids slowly. Noncaloric fluids include water, instant broth, diet drinks, sugar-free tea/coffee, ice chips, sugar-free ice Popsicle, and sugar-free gelatin.
- Replace carbohydrate in diet with fluid equivalents. Consume 10–15 grams of carbohydrate every 1–2 hours. Substitutions include 1/2 cup

fruit juice or fruit drink, 1/2 cup regular gelatin, 1/2–3/4 cup regular sodas, 1 regular double ice Popsicle, 1 fruit juice ice Popsicle, 1/4 cup sherbet, 1 cup soup, 1 cup milk, 1/4 cup regular pudding, 1/2 cup sugar-free pudding, or 1/2 cup ice cream.

- When the person is able to tolerate solid food, suggest small, frequent amounts of food containing 10–15 grams carbohydrate, including 1/2 cup cooked cereal, 1/2 cup mashed potatoes, 1/3 cup rice, 1 slice bread/toast, 3 graham cracker halves, 6 saltine crackers, and 6 vanilla wafers.

For minor illness and stress, a temporary increase in both the basal and bolus insulin doses may be necessary, as well as an increase in the insulin:carbohydrate ratio and ISF. It's best to increase doses gradually based on frequent SMBG results. With MDI and CSII, meal bolus doses can be calculated based on actual intake and given postmeal to prevent hypoglycemia.

CHAPTER SIX

Access to Diabetes Educators/Registered Dietitians

For more information on providing and accessing quality diabetes care and education:

- **Contact an ADA Recognized Education Program.** About 1,300 programs have achieved Education Recognition. The National Standards for Diabetes Self-Management Education require that an RD be a member of the instructional team (23). To locate a Recognized program in your area, call 1-800-DIABETES (1-800-342-2383) or visit the ADA website at *www.diabetes.org/education/edustate2.asp.*
- **Contact the American Association of Diabetes Educators (AADE).** To contact an AADE member in your area (located by zip code), call 1-800-TEAMUP4 (1-800-832-6874) or visit the AADE website at *www.aadenet.org* and look under "find an educator."
- **Contact a local endocrinology practice.** These may employ or have access to one or more diabetes educators. There may be diabetes education programs at a local hospital or affiliated with a large group medical practice to which people can be referred.

References

1. Diabetes Control and Complications Trial Research Group: The effect of intensive treatment of diabetes on the development and progression of long-term complications in insulin-dependent diabetes mellitus. *N Engl J Med* 329:977–86, 1993

2. UK Prospective Diabetes Study Group: Intensive blood-glucose control with sulphonylureas or insulin compared with conventional treatment and risk of complications in patients with type 2 diabetes (UKPDS 33). *Lancet* 352: 837–53, 1998

3. Diabetes Control and Complications Trial Research Group: Nutrition interventions for intensive therapy in the Diabetes Control and Complications Trial. *J Am Diet Assoc* 93:768–72, 1993

4. American Diabetes Association: Nutrition recommendations for people with diabetes mellitus (Position Statement). *Diabetes Care* 24 (Suppl. 1): S45–47, 2001

5. American Diabetes Association: Postprandial blood glucose (Consensus Statement). *Diabetes Care* 24:775–78, 2001

6. Laredo R: Carbohydrate counting for children and adolescents. *Diabetes Spectrum* 13:149–52, 2000

7. Reader D: Carbohydrate counting for pregnant women. *Diabetes Spectrum* 13:152–53, 2000

8. Albright A: Carbohydrate counting for athletes. *Diabetes Spectrum* 13:154–56, 2000

9. Johnson MA: Carbohydrate counting for people with type 2 diabetes. *Diabetes Spectrum* 13:156–58, 2000

10. Saffel-Shrier S: Carbohydrate counting for older patients. *Diabetes Spectrum* 13:158–62, 2000

11. Paddock BW: Carbohydrate counting in institutions. *Diabetes Spectrum* 13:162–64, 2000

12. Holler H, Pastors J: Process of diabetes medical nutrition therapy. In *Diabetes Medical Nutrition Therapy.* Chicago, IL: American Dietetic Association, and Alexandria, VA: American Diabetes Association, 1997

13. Diabetes Care and Education Dietetic Practice Group: Scope of practice for qualified dietetics professionals in diabetes care and education. *J Am Diet Assoc* 100(10):1205–207, 2000

14. Graff MR, Gross TM, Juth SE, Charlson J: How well are individuals on intensive insulin therapy counting carbohydrates (Abstract)? Presented at the 2000 International Diabetes Federation Meeting, Mexico City

15. Warshaw HS, Powers MA: A search for answers about foods with polyols (sugar alcohols). *Diabetes Educator* 25(3):307–21, 1999

16. American Diabetes Association: *Intensive Diabetes Management.* 2nd ed. Alexandria, VA: American Diabetes Association, 1998, p. 75

17. Franz MJ, Bantle JP (Eds.): *American Diabetes Association Guide to Medical Nutrition Therapy for Diabetes.* Alexandria, VA: American Diabetes Association, 1999

18. Walsh PA, Roberts R: *Pumping Insulin.* 3rd ed. San Diego, CA: Torrey Pines Press, 2000

19. Ahern JA, Gatcomb PM, Held NA, Petit WA, Tamborlane WV: Exaggerated hyperglycemia after a pizza meal in well-controlled diabetes. *Diabetes Care* 16:578–80, 1993

20. Foster-Powell K, Brand-Miller J: International tables of glycemic index. *Am J Clin Nutr* 62:871S–893S, 1995

21. Diabetes Control and Complications Trial Research Group: Weight gain associated with intensive therapy in the Diabetes Control and Complications Trial. *Diabetes Care* 11:67–73, 1997

22. Gillespie SJ, Kulkarni KD, Daly AE: Using carbohydrate counting in diabetes clinical practice. *J Am Diet Assoc* 98(8):897-905, 1998

23. American Diabetes Association: National standards for diabetes self-management education (Position Statement). *Diabetes Care* 24 (Suppl. 1): S126–33, 2001

APPENDIX 1: Glycemic Control for People with Diabetes

	Normal	Goal	Additional Action Suggested
Whole blood values			
Average preprandial glucose (mg/dl)	<100	80–120	<80/>140
Average bedtime glucose (mg/dl)	<110	100–140	<100/>160
2 hours after start of meals (mg/dl)		160–180*	
Plasma values			
Average preprandial glucose (mg/dl)	<100	90–130	<90/>150
Average bedtime glucose (mg/dl)	<120	110–150	<110/>180
2 hours after start of meals (mg/dl)		170–190*	
Hemoglobin A_{1c} (HbA$_{1c}$) (%)	<6	<7	>8

*These recommendations come from consensus among diabetes care providers. No ADA recommendation exists for postprandial glucose levels (American Diabetes Association: Postprandial blood glucose. *Diabetes Care* 24:775–78, 2001).

These values are by necessity generalized to the entire population of individuals with diabetes and are for nonpregnant adults. Patients with comorbid disease, the very young and older adults, and others with unusual conditions or circumstances may warrant different treatment goals. "Additional action suggested" depends on individual patient circumstances. Such actions may include enhanced diabetes self-management education, comanagement with a diabetes team, referral to an endocrinologist, change in pharmacological therapy, initiation of or increase in SMBG, or more frequent contact with the patient. HbA$_{1c}$ is referenced to a nondiabetic range of 4–6%.

APPENDIX 2 :   How Much Carbohydrate to Eat and When?

Calorie Range:
Carbohydrate Grams:
Carbohydrate Servings:

Breakfast	Sample Meal	Sample Meal
Carbohydrate Grams	_____	_____
Carbohydrate Servings	_____	_____

Lunch	Sample Meal	Sample Meal
Carbohydrate Grams	_____	_____
Carbohydrate Servings	_____	_____

Snack	Sample Snack	Sample Snack
Carbohydrate Grams	_____	_____
Carbohydrate Servings	_____	_____

Dinner	Sample Meal	Sample Meal
Carbohydrate Grams	_____	_____
Carbohydrate Servings	_____	_____

Snack		
Carbohydrate Grams	_____	_____
Carbohydrate Servings	_____	_____

Notes: _____
_____
_____
_____
_____
_____
_____
_____
_____
_____
_____
_____
_____
_____

APPENDIX 3 : Carbohydrate Counting Resources

Nutrition Facts (food label)

The total carbohydrate listed on the Nutrition Facts label is the most readily accessible and most accurate source of carbohydrate information. Note "total carbohydrate grams." Do not count the grams of sugars—these are included in total carbohydrate grams.

Books

Warshaw HS, Kulkarni K: *Complete Guide to Carb Counting.* Alexandria, VA, American Diabetes Association, 2001

Holzmeister L: *The Diabetes Carbohydrate and Fat Gram Guide.* 2nd ed. Alexandria, VA, American Diabetes Association, 2000

Holzmeister L: *Complete Guide to Convenience Food Counts.* Alexandria, VA, American Diabetes Association, 2001

The Official Pocket Guide to Diabetic Exchanges. Alexandria, VA, American Diabetes Association, and Chicago, IL, American Dietetic Association, 1997

Netzer CT: *The Complete Book of Food Counts.* 5th ed. Dell Publishing, 2000

Netzer CT: *The Corinne T. Netzer Carbohydrate Counter.* 2nd ed. Dell Publishing, 1998

Kraus B, Reilly-Pardo M: *Calories and Carbohydrates.* 14th ed. Signet, 2001

Pennington J: *Bowes and Church Food Values of Portions Commonly Used.* 17th ed. Lippincott, 1998

Borushek A:*The Doctor's Pocket Calorie, Fat & Carbohydrate Counter.* Family Health Publisher, 2000

Restaurant Information

Warshaw HS, Blackburn G: *American Diabetes Association Guide to Healthy Restaurant Eating.* Alexandria, VA, American Diabetes Association, 1998

Licthen J: *Dining Lean: How to Eat Healthy in Your Favorite Restaurants.* Houston, TX, Nutrifit Publishing, 2000

Natow AB, Heslin J-A: *Eating Out Food Counter: Restaurant, Takeout, and Snack Foods.* Pocket Books, 1998

Warshaw HS: *The Restaurant Companion: A Guide to Healthier Restaurant Eating.* Chicago, Surrey Books, 1999

APPENDIX 3: Carbohydrate Counting Resources (continued)

Diabetes Forecast: Healthy Chain Restaurant Eating (monthly column)

Ethnic and Regional Food Practices: A Series. Alexandria, VA, American Diabetes Association; Chicago, IL, American Dietetic Association, www.eatright.org/catalog/diabetes.html

Nutrition in the Fast Lane: The Fast Food Dining Guide. Indianapolis, IN, Franklin Publishing, 2001

Chain restaurant web sites: Review carbohydrate and other nutrients for these offerings

Cookbooks

All cookbooks for people with diabetes published by the American Diabetes Association and other publishers. Carbohydrate information is provided per serving. Order books published by American Diabetes Association from 800-ADA-ORDER (232-6733) or on the Internet at www.store.org.

Internet

www.cyberdiet.com has a database of thousands foods with carbohydrate content as well as other nutrients.

www.usda.gov/fnic/foodcomp is the site for the United States Department of Agriculture (USDA) nutrient database. (This nutrient database is the base of many commercial databases.) This database can be downloaded. A program allowing you to search the database is also available. The database is also available on CD-ROM and may be purchased from the Government Printing Office

www.eNASCO.com is an online catalog of nutrition teaching resources, food models, and scales, among other items.

www.diabetesnet.com offers diabetes resources, including food scales.

Commercial Software

Many commercial software programs are available that provide you with a nutrition database of commonly eaten foods. Make sure the one you purchase contains a sizable number of foods, at least 15,000, and includes the types of foods you eat.

www.healthetech.com: inexpensive software for PDAs.

APPENDIX 4: Record Keeping Form

Carbohydrate Counting and Blood Glucose Record

Day/date _____

Time/ meal	Diabetes medicines			Food		Carb count (choices/ grams)	Blood glucose checks							
	Type	Bolus amount	Correction amount	Type	Amount		Fasting/ before break-fast	After break-fast	Before lunch	After lunch	Before dinner	After dinner	Before bed	Other

Notes about day:

APPENDIX 5: Carbohydrate Counting Teaching Checklist

**Basic Carbohydrate
Counting Skills:***

- ☐ Understand benefits of carbohydrate counting
- ☐ Know what foods contain carbohydrate
- ☐ Understand that carbohydrate-containing foods are part of a healthy diet
- ☐ Understand ADA guidelines about eating sweets
- ☐ Measure a serving of carbohydrate
- ☐ Count servings or choices or grams
- ☐ Know how to divide carbohydrate into meals and snacks
- ☐ Understand portion control
- ☐ Use portion control equipment: food label, measuring equipment, eyes
- ☐ Have and use resources listing for carbohydrate counts
- ☐ Know general guidelines for protein and fat

**Advanced Carbohydrate
Counting Skills:***

- ☐ Mastery of all basic carbohydrate counting concepts
- ☐ Understand insulin action
- ☐ Understand insulin regulation for 24-hour blood glucose control
- ☐ Explain background or basal and food coverage or bolus insulin
- ☐ Calculate insulin:carbohydrate ratio
- ☐ Calculate insulin sensitivity factor and correction or supplemental doses
- ☐ Determine premeal insulin doses
- ☐ Explain pattern management
- ☐ Correct hyperglycemia
- ☐ Correct hypoglycemia
- ☐ Count carbohydrate and adjust insulin for special situations:
  - ☐ High-protein and/or high-fat meals
  - ☐ Foods containing fiber
  - ☐ To minimize weight gain with improved glycemic control
  - ☐ Restaurant foods
  - ☐ Meals on vacations and holidays and in other people's homes
  - ☐ Alcohol use
  - ☐ Physical activity and exercise
  - ☐ Sick days and stress

*All people with diabetes should know their individual target blood glucose levels, target hemoglobin A1c, and the points at which to take action. If their postprandial glucose (PPG) levels will be monitored, they also should know their target PPGs.

A P P E N D I X 6 : How Much Carbohydrate Is Needed?

	Desire weight loss*	Many older women	Women, older adults	Larger women, older men	Children, teen girls, active	Teen boys, active men
Calorie level	About 1200	About 1400	About 1600	About 1800	About 2200	About 2800
Calorie range	1200–1500	1300–1600	1400–1700	1600–1900	1800–2300	2200–2800
Carbohydrate grams	180	180	195	210	240	300
Carbohydrate choices	12	12	12–13	13–14	15–16	18–20
Grains, beans and starchy vegetables	6	6	6	7	9	11
Vegetables†	3	3	3	4	4	5
Fruits	3	3	3	3	3	4
Milk‡	2	2	2–3	2–3	2–3	2–3
Meats	2 (4 oz)	2 (4 oz)	2 (5 oz)	2 (5 oz)	2 (6 ox)	3 (7 oz)
Fat g/servings (based on 30% of calories)	40/4	47/5	54/6	60/7	74/9	93/12

Chart adapted from Diabetes Meal Planning Made Easy, 2nd ed. American Diabetes Association. 2000.
*Some older women and men who are small in stature and sedentary may need to eat no more than 1200 calories to lose weight. At 1200 calories, a person may need a vitamin and mineral supplement that provides 100% of the Daily Value to meet nutrition needs.
†Three vegetables equals 15 grams carbohydrate or 1 carb choice.
‡Teenagers, young adults to age 24, women who are pregnant or breastfeeding, and adults older than 50 need 1200 mg of calcium each day. Adults younger than 50 need 1000 mg of calcium per day. Some people may require calcium supplementation. Each cup of milk or yogurt contains about 300 mg of calcium. Each serving of milk is equivalent to about 12 grams of carbohydrate or roughly 1 carbohydrate choice.

Index

Alcohol, 1, 30, 31, 45

Carbohydrate
    calculating needs, 8–11, 57
    servings, 7, 11
Children, 3
Continuous subcutaneous insulin
    infusion (CSII), 2, 3, 10, 21,
    37–41
Correction dose, 29, 37

Diabetes Control and Complications
    Trial (DCCT), 1
Diabetes medical nutrition therapy, 4

1800 rule, 28
Elderly, 3
Ethnic foods, 45
Exercise, 31, 37, 46

Fat, 14, 31, 38, 42
Fiber, 38, 43
1500 rule, 28–29

Gastroparesis, 30, 31, 38
Glycemic control
    recommendations, 51
Glycemic index, 38, 43

Hyperglycemia, correcting, 30–31
Hypoglycemia, correcting, 31–32

Insulin
    action, 22
    delivery, 23–25
    dose, 26
    pumps, 37–41
    regimens, 22–25
    sensitivity, 26
    supplemental dose, 29
    timing, 30–31
Insulin:carbohydrate ratio
    calculating, 26–28, 37
Insulin sensitivity factor, 28

Multiple daily injection (MDI), 2, 3,
    10, 21

Nutrients, 9
Nutrition facts, 3, 5, 8, 13–14

Pattern management, 30
Polyols, 13–14
Portions, 11–12
Postprandial blood glucose (PPG),
    1, 51
Protein, 14, 31, 38, 42

Record keeping form, 55
Restaurant eating, 7, 38, 44–45
Rule of 15, 32
Rule of 500, 27–28

Servings
    food label, 8
    diabetes, 8
    vs. grams, 11

Sick days, 30, 38, 46–47
Snacks, 10
Stress, 30, 46–47
Supplemental dose, 29
Sweets, 7, 9

Teaching
    checklist, 56
    tools, 5

United Kingdom Prospective
    Diabetes Study, 1

Weight gain, 32, 43–44

About the American Diabetes Association

The American Diabetes Association is the nation's leading voluntary health organization supporting diabetes research, information, and advocacy. Its mission is to prevent and cure diabetes and to improve the lives of all people affected by diabetes. The American Diabetes Association is the leading publisher of comprehensive diabetes information. Its huge library of practical and authoritative books for people with diabetes covers every aspect of self-care—cooking and nutrition, fitness, weight control, medications, complications, emotional issues, and general self-care.

To order American Diabetes Association books: Call 1-800-232-6733. http://store.diabetes.org [Note: there is no need to use **www** when typing this particular Web address]

To join the American Diabetes Association: Call 1-800-806-7801. www.diabetes.org/membership

For more information about diabetes or ADA programs and services: Call 1-800-342-2383. E-mail: Customerservice@diabetes.org www.diabetes.org

To locate an ADA/NCQA Recognized Provider of quality diabetes care in your area: Call 1-703-549-1500 ext. 2202. www.diabetes.org/recognition/Physicians/ListAll.asp

To find an ADA Recognized Education Program in your area: Call 1-888-232-0822. www.diabetes.org/recognition/education.asp

To join the fight to increase funding for diabetes research, end discrimination, and improve insurance coverage: Call 1-800-342-2383. www.diabetes.org/advocacy

To find out how you can get involved with the programs in your community: Call 1-800-342-2383. See below for program Web addresses.

- *American Diabetes Month:* Educational activities aimed at those diagnosed with diabetes—month of November. www.diabetes.org/ADM
- *American Diabetes Alert:* Annual public awareness campaign to find the undiagnosed—held the fourth Tuesday in March. www.diabetes.org/alert
- *The Diabetes Assistance & Resources Program (DAR):* diabetes awareness program targeted to the Latino community. www.diabetes.org/DAR
- *African American Program:* diabetes awareness program targeted to the African American community. www.diabetes.org/africanamerican
- *Awakening the Spirit: Pathways to Diabetes Prevention & Control:* diabetes awareness program targeted to the Native American community. www.diabetes.org/awakening

To find out about an important research project regarding type 2 diabetes: www.diabetes.org/ada/research.asp

To obtain information on making a planned gift or charitable bequest: Call 1-888-700-7029. www.diabetes.org/ada/plan.asp

To make a donation or memorial contribution: Call 1-800-342-2383. www.diabetes.org/ada/cont.asp